I0428371

100 things I learned from my elders

Having Sex over age70 is like shooting pool with a rope

Life is like a boomerang
Everything you throw out
comes back to you

Everyday tell your family that you love them

With exception to a house and a car pay cash for everything

Friends come and go but family is always here for you

I have found that I feel the wealthiest when I live my life in the most simple fashion

Every day look in the mirror and tell yourself it's going to be a great day!

People always ask me how I have such a great relationship with my kids, One of the most important items is telling them that I love them every day!

The secret to my success is to be thankful for my health and laugh a lot.

Never blame if you want to be successful, A poor milkman blames the cow

Always to the right thing, even when nobody is looking!

I have learned that the best way to have a good night sleep is to never go to bed angry

Life has been amazing, I have learned that everything I give (love, money, help) always comes back to me multiplied

With Kids, remember it might seem tough when they are young but they will soon be older and not even around so cherish every minute!

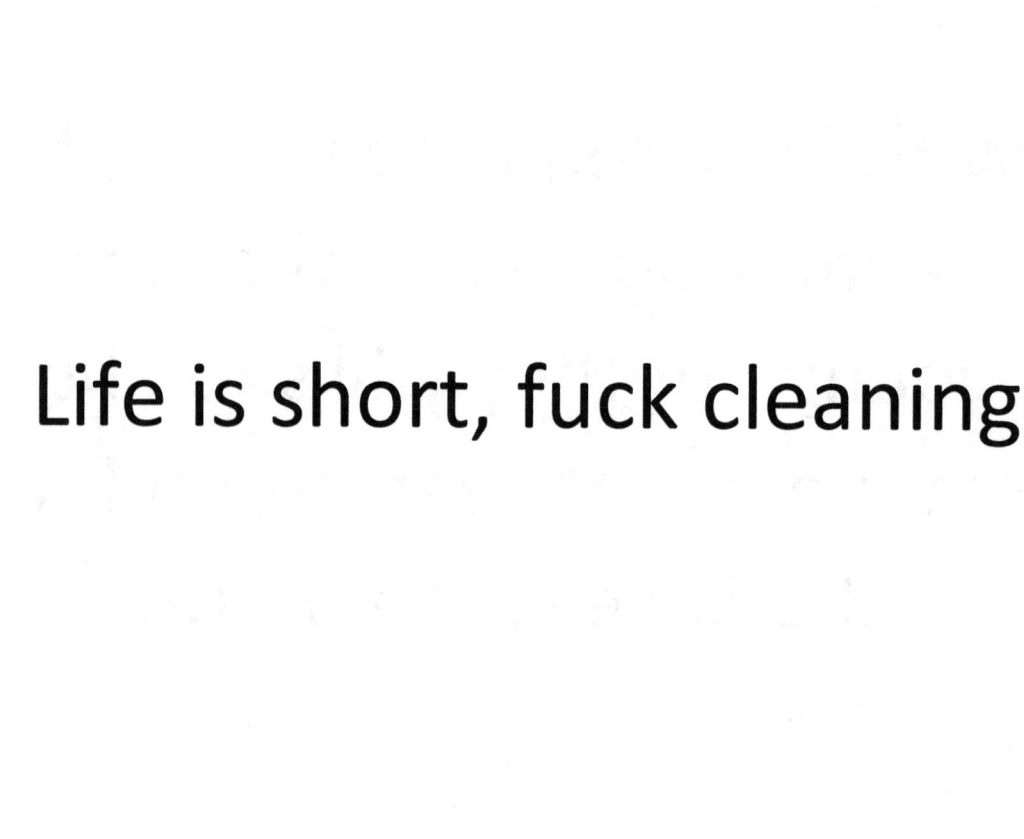

Life is short, fuck cleaning

Seek out the humor in everything

In order to achieve your goals (personal or professional) you must ignite yourself on fire!

Luck is really an acronym and it stands for Learning Under Correct Knowledge

Remember in business, the better we treat each other internally the better we treat our clients

Mr. B always says the secret to his happiness is to never grow up, always be like a kid

You really need to watch who you hang out with, you are the average of the few people you hang out with the most.

Sometimes in life you need to turn chicken shit into chicken salad.

Remember, if you work and prepare hard enough then there is no pressure!

When giving a speech remember that you need to stop talking before people stop listening!

To be successful stop looking at where you are at and always look where you want to go! Picture the end result

Life is short
Fuck Cleaning

I go to bed each night at piece, I never go to be angry at anyone

People always ask me how we had a successful marriage and I always tell them that I put Marriage #1, nothing else gets in our way

Don't worry about the little things, I try to laugh at everything

If I could give any advice about your career it would be absolutely to follow your dreams and do what you love. It really can happen

Remember that everyday is a gift, who are you going to help today

I try to do something everyday for myself.

I really believe that honesty is one my best qualities. It helps me sleep well

My best advice is to walk or do something everything day to exercise. Over the last 90 years this has kept me healthy and happy!

My best advice is to have a dog or cat, their love is forever healing

Remember, it's really up to you each day to choose to be happy and healthy.

Choose your thoughts wisely, it really does make a difference each day

At an early age I learned that its hard to be unhappy when you are exercising. I try and do something every day!

Travel when you can, before you know it you will be old like me and the memories are what count.

My secret to happiness is giving thanks every morning I get up. I try to think of 3 things to genuinely be thankful for!

After all these years, I think I'm still around for having Margaritas every Friday with my friends!

When I hit 80 I really stopped worrying about anything. I try to laugh a lot and I have good friends!

My best advice for money is to never get into too much debt and my advice for happiness is to be loving every day to anyone you meet.

My long life of happiness comes from giving. I try to give back every day to someone.

Try every morning to read a positive book or magazine!

I had a man once tell me this stuff like honey from New Zealand (Manuka) was best for my health. Every day I have it on my toast!

I saw a tombstone 50 years ago that said I came, I saw, I gave in Latin and I had tried to live like that!

One thing that has helped me live so long is just being out in the sunshine. I get at least 15 minutes every day and I'm happy.

I'm always learning, I think that's why I am still here.

I try to read the comics every weekend!

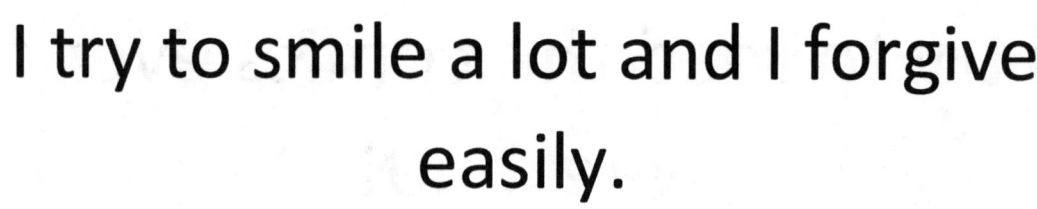

I try to smile a lot and I forgive easily.

I stay active and when I can I always take the stairs!

I recommend pets, my dog has really helped me over the years!

I try to go camping at least once a year. Even at 90 years old I appreciate the simple things.

Every Saturday I read by this little stream by my house. I sit and just look at the sky and give thanks.

My father told me a long time ago to always do the right thing, even when nobody is looking.

I try to take a nap every day, I still keep busy but I like to rest.

I tell my grandson knock knock jokes! He laughs just as much as I do

The smartest thing I did when I was young was figure out something that I loved. I loved animals and became a veterinarian.

I try to do something interesting or new every day, it keeps me young!

I try to tell at least 3 people per day that I appreciate them.

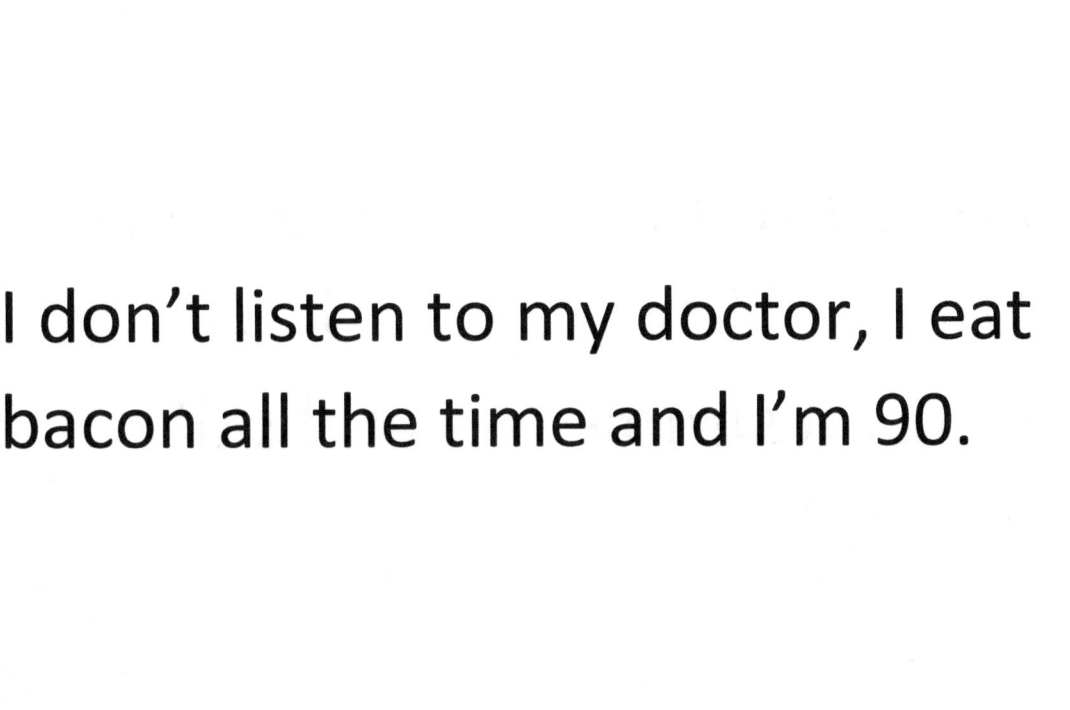

I don't listen to my doctor, I eat bacon all the time and I'm 90.

People ask me all the time why am I so happy, really I just enjoy a simple life and putz around.

I think I'm still here because I eat healthy and I have a family that loves me.

I was in prisoner work camp in World War II. I had to sleep outside in a hole so I don't complain much.

Remember that in business your internal customers are just as important.

I like to sing every day, I feel alive when I sing!

After all these years I think having a shot of whiskey with my cousin every Saturday has kept me here!

Try and travel before you have kids!

I think my Dad told me once a Bird in the hand is better than two in the bushes. I now know he was right.

My best advice for your marriage is to remember when you are in a heated argument that the objective is not to win but to make progress.

I try to seek the humor in everything!

Life is short, try to celebrate every little success!

I once asked a man about borrowing his RV, he told me that RV's are like puppies, you don't loan them out!

I eat liver and onions every couple months!

Try to Meditate as much as possible

Feed your mind like you feed your body! I try every day

My best advice is hard work at anything. This has always proven successful in my marriage, finances, and everything.

To be successful in business remember the story of "Lagniappe"

To be successful in life put your marriage and your kids first everything else comes after.

My advice is take as many videos and pictures as you can. It goes quick.

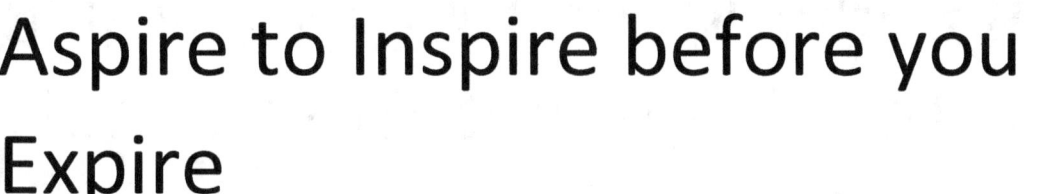

Aspire to Inspire before you Expire

Remember that when working with a Team that Trust is the foundation!

Now more than ever focus on the first 15% and the rest will follow

To be successful, always ask yourself "What is the best use of my time right now?"

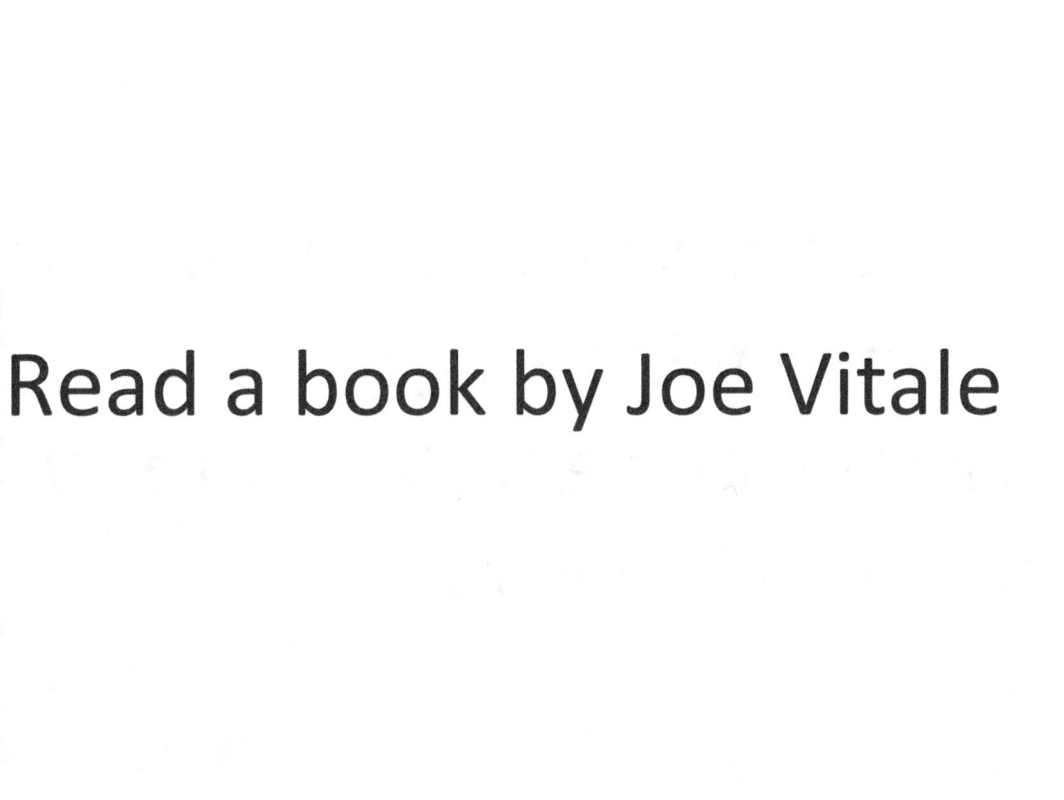
Read a book by Joe Vitale

If you really want to know how you are doing ask your customer on a scale of 1 to 10 how would you rank us?

Remember if you want something done that action creates action. Get up and do something

Pay off your credit card each month! I will give you great sense of mind

Don't compare your life to others, you are on your own journey

Remember that your children only get one childhood

Remember Mark Twain " Eat the ugliest frog first"

Remember to focus on your most important goal, if you chase two rabbits you won't catch either one!

A wise woman once told me that she believed to her core that life should be lived abundantly!

Be clear why you are here,
purpose is everything

Remember that all blame is a waste of time

Try to follow W. Clement Stone's example of "everyone is out there trying to help me"

Remember that your enthusiasm with anything in life is contagious!

You must approach all of your training with a positive mental attitude! You will succeed!

www.ingramcontent.com/pod-product-compliance
Lightning Source LLC
Chambersburg PA
CBHW070549290526
45790CB00002B/618

* 9 7 8 1 5 0 3 1 0 8 2 5 7 *